Vinicius Pedrazzi
Cássio do Nascimento
Gizele V. B. Pedrazzi

Necessary precautions for disinfecting toothbrushes

Vinicius Pedrazzi
Cássio do Nascimento
Gizele V. B. Pedrazzi

Necessary precautions for disinfecting toothbrushes

Decontaminating toothbrushes

ScienciaScripts

Imprint
Any brand names and product names mentioned in this book are subject to trademark, brand or patent protection and are trademarks or registered trademarks of their respective holders. The use of brand names, product names, common names, trade names, product descriptions etc. even without a particular marking in this work is in no way to be construed to mean that such names may be regarded as unrestricted in respect of trademark and brand protection legislation and could thus be used by anyone.

Cover image: www.ingimage.com

This book is a translation from the original published under ISBN 978-613-9-67988-1.

Publisher:
Sciencia Scripts
is a trademark of
Dodo Books Indian Ocean Ltd. and OmniScriptum S.R.L publishing group

120 High Road, East Finchley, London, N2 9ED, United Kingdom
Str. Armeneasca 28/1, office 1, Chisinau MD-2012, Republic of Moldova, Europe
Printed at: see last page
ISBN: 978-620-8-19137-5

SUMMARY

1 INTRODUCTION

The concepts of oral health and systemic health should not, at first, be interpreted as separate entities. Oral health is integrated with systemic health, and this information encourages the important consideration that oral health means much more than healthy teeth, and that a human being cannot be considered healthy without good oral health conditions.

Significant progress has been made in oral health, but there is still a lot of work to be done. There are safe and effective preventive measures that everyone can take to improve their health, and dental surgeons play a key role in disseminating prevention information, especially about the most prevalent oral diseases, i.e. dental caries and periodontal disease.

Dental researchers have been trying to understand the microbial nature of oral infections for the past 120 years. The view of plaque and its constituent microorganisms has changed from the specific plaque theory to the non-specific plaque theory, and then again to the theory of the presence of specific pathogens in plaque (OVERMAN, 2000).

Dental plaque has currently been described as an example of a biofilm. Biofilms are ubiquitous, and are defined as communities of bacteria adhered to a surface, embedded in an extracellular matrix of host and bacterial polymers. The properties of bacteria change markedly when they grow in a biofilm, and this can be of major clinical relevance, since bacteria present in biofilms have an increased resistance to antimicrobial agents (OVERMAN, 2000, MARSH, 2004; TEN CATE, 2006).

These new concepts have gained fundamental importance in the new therapies to be applied for the removal and/or control of periodontal biofilm, and thus for the prevention of oral diseases and any systemic repercussions arising from them.

The use of instruments for routine mechanical cleaning of teeth dates back thousands of years. Kauffman, (1924); Kanner, (1926); Pader, (1988), reported the practice of preventive oral hygiene measures by the Egyptians, Sumerians and Babylonians around 3,000 years before Christ.

There is controversy over the exact origin of toothbrushes. It is believed that the toothbrush as it is known today, with bristles perpendicular to the handle, was invented by the Chinese (McCauley, 1946; Ring, 1985; Bogopolsky, 1995), probably around 1490 (Ring, 1985) and, over time, has undergone various modifications in order to improve its quality and function, as can be seen from the diversity of models available on the market.

For a long time, toothbrush bristles were of animal origin (pig or wild boar hair - the latter being the best). Today, it's easy to understand the great risk these bristles posed because they lacked standardization, had a high water sorption capacity (>90%) and were a risk of zoonoses. They only began to be replaced in 1938, with the introduction of nylon, but their use, however, only became completely widespread after 1950, when DuPont® improved the manufacture of bristles with a technology that produced fine filaments with rounded ends (GOLDING, 1982; PADER, 1988).

The filaments of modern brushes are almost universally made of nylon, and the best variety of nylon is known as 6.12, where one tuft can support adjacent ones, an effect that is more pronounced in so-called multi-tuft brushes, with tufts arranged so that they are very close together.

These data show that the use of toothbrushes as preventive dental material for oral hygiene is not a recent practice. However, the vast majority of people do not take any special care with this instrument, either in choosing it or in the hygienic care related to it. Samson (1972) in his article on oral hygiene and the use of toothbrushes in the United Kingdom, cited cases of collective use of the toothbrush by the whole family and situations where it was used for something other than the purpose for which it was created.

The human oral cavity comprises a complex and heterogeneous ecosystem, including soft and hard tissues and fluids, which are colonized by various species of microorganisms (TAKAHASHI, 2005; TAWAKOLI et at. 2013). In addition to high diversity, the oral ecosystem is characterized by constant transitions over time, which are influenced by various factors, including external disturbances (such as the presence of food debris as a result of the chewing process, mechanical oral hygiene, antimicrobial solutions, antibiotics, food), intra-biogeographical differences (such as hard or soft tissues), interaction with the host and secretions (KOLENBRANDER et al., 2010; NIKITKOVA, 2013).

The interaction between these factors can favor the colonization and proliferation of microorganisms on oral surfaces, predicting transitions from health to disease in the oral cavity. Saliva can also be considered an important source of nutrients and is essential for the formation of maturing oral biofilm. Many salivary components (such as proteins) can promote microbial adhesion on surfaces and can cause aggregation of oral microorganisms, resulting in the enlargement of the oral cavity (KOLENBRANDER et al., 2010).

More than 700 microbial species, including fungi, viruses and unclassified microorganisms, can be found colonizing the different surfaces of the oral cavity (NIKITKOVA, 2013; XU X et al., 2014). Most of them are commensal species and are beneficial in promoting oral health (NIKITKOVA, 2013). However, some of these species, under specific conditions, are able to overcome the host's protective responses and have been implicated in oral diseases, and are referred to as pathogenic species.

Disruption of the balance of the oral microbiota, resulting in an overload of pathogenic species, can cause caries, periodontitis and stomatitis, which are among the most common oral microbial infections in humans. *Streptococcus spp*. and *Actinomyces spp*. are pioneer colonizers, abundant and commonly related to supragingival plaque in the initial phase of biofilm formation (KOLENBRANDER, 2000). They can acidify the oral biofilm, increasing its cariogenic potential (TAKAHASHI, 2005; KOLENBRANDER, 2000).

After the biofilm matures, anaerobic and proteolytic bacteria such as *Porphyromonas gingivalis, Tanerella forsythia, Treponema denticola and Fusobacterium spp.* are often found harboring the subgingival biofilm (KOWALSKI & GÓRSKA, 2014). Bacterial proteases and the metabolic products for their lysis have the potential to induce host responses such as inflammation and immunoreactions, leading to periodontitis/peri-implantitis (MAYANAGI et al, 2004; GOHLER et al., 2014). *Candida spp.* are the most common fungi in the oral cavity and are strongly associated with denture stomatitis (GENDREAU & LOEWY, 2011; IȘERI et al., 2011). In addition, they have been detected as an opportunistic species in periodontal and peri-implant lesions (LEONHARDT et al., 2003).

The mechanical removal of formed oral biofilm (including toothbrush, dental floss and tongue scrapers) is considered the most effective method of oral hygiene of soft and hard tissues, significantly reducing the microbial count in the oral cavity (RAMAGE et al., 2010; CROCOMBE et al., 2012). In addition, complementary hygiene methods using mouthwashes and topical fluoride help to remove remaining debris and prevent/minimize microbial adhesion on oral surfaces (TEN CATE & MARSH, 1994; Gupta et al., 2014).

However, a major concern to be overcome in dentistry is the contamination of toothbrushes by microorganisms after brushing, with consequent infection of oral tissues. Toothbrush bristles are colonized by various species of microorganisms after use, and the viability of these species has been reported to vary from one day to one week (SPOLIDORIO et al., 2003; FRAZELLE & MUNRO, 2012). Food debris on the bristles acting as nutrients and their exposure to contaminated aerosols (i.e. storage in toilets) can precipitate and facilitate the growth and proliferation of various species (FRAZELLE & MUNRO, 2012; TAJI & ROGERS, 1998).

Several investigations have reported toothbrushes contaminated by non-pathogenic and/or pathogenic species, with a relevant impact on the development and proliferation of oral diseases (GLASS, 1992; BALAPPANAVAR et al., 2009; RATSON et al., 2012).

In addition, this condition can contribute to the worsening of systemic diseases, including respiratory and cardiovascular problems and sepsis (OLIVEIRA et al., 2014).

The disinfection of toothbrushes is a subject that has received little attention from researchers, despite the fact that it is known that they can be contaminated by microorganisms associated with various bacterial diseases in the oral cavity, such as dental caries (Svanberg, 1978), periodontal disease (Pinto et al...) or others caused by fungi and even sporulated, more resistant forms (MARCANO, 1981; NELSON-FON et al., 2000; SATO et al., 1997), 1997) or others caused by fungi and even viruses and sporulated, more resistant forms (MARCANO, 1981; NELSON-FILHO et al., 2000; SATO et al., 2004).

The literature also shows that simple routine hygiene with a toothbrush can cause bacteremia (SCONYERS et al. 1973; SATO et al., 2005). Thus, the toothbrush, which not only helps to remove dental biofilm but also massages the gums, favoring tissue exchange in the gingival sulcus, could indirectly lead to the onset of a disease due to the bacteremia that would follow brushing.

The presence of microorganisms on toothbrushes used by 20 healthy individuals was evaluated by Caudry et al. (1995). The authors also evaluated antiseptic mouthwashes (Virkon®, Listerine®, Cepacol®, Scope® and Plax®) for their bactericidal power on conventional and interdental brushes, concluding that immersing the brush heads in Listerine (essential oils) for 20 minutes after brushing was sufficient to eliminate bacterial contamination.

Meier et al., 1996 tested cetylpyridinium chloride (CCP), a quaternary ammonium compound, as an alternative to eliminate residual microorganisms in air-dried brushes packed in travel cases. Strains *of Staphylococcus epidermidis* or *Candida albicans* were inoculated onto the bristles and when sprayed with CCP (half the sample), there was a 100% reduction for bacteria and 94% for fungi, proving to be a practical and efficient method for disinfecting travel brushes.

Due to the risk of possible contamination of toothbrushes, which could lead to cross-infection or even re-infection, some researchers have focused their studies on this subject, with highly significant results, using both bis-biguanide (chlorhexidine digluconate) and cetylpyridinium chloride in the form of sprays (SATO et al., 2004; SATO et al, 2005).

In a recent clinical study carried out by Mehta et al. (2007), which microbiologically evaluated the extent of contamination of toothbrushes after use and storage of the brush heads with a plastic cover, and the effectiveness of chlorhexidine and essential oils in decontaminating them, they found exuberant contamination in 70% of the brushes evaluated. The use of plastic protectors led to the growth of opportunistic microorganisms such as *Pseudomonas aeruginosa*. Immersing the brushes in chlorhexidine gluconate solution (0.2%) proved to be the most effective in bacterial decontamination.

There is now a consensus that toothbrush disinfection is a key step in oral hygiene. Many studies have evaluated various toothbrush disinfection protocols, including immersion/spray in different disinfectant solutions or mouthwashes, and bristles impregnated with antimicrobial agents (SATO et al., 2005; AL-AHMAD et al., 2010; do NASCIMENTO et al., 2014).

Most of these protocols have been shown to be effective in reducing microbial colonization on bristles. However, most of these investigations used culture-dependent methods for microbial assessment, in which only viable cells could be detected. Using culture-independent methods (i.e. genetic material), we can detect and identify viable and non-viable microorganisms.

Thus, the final detection result may differ depending on the method used. Considering that microbial cell death can occur due to the absence of a significant amount of nutrients and/or microbial competition during the storage of toothbrushes, and the products of cell lysis and degradation can interfere with the inflammatory process of oral tissues, we proposed two randomized crossover studies in controlled clinical investigations identifying and quantifying, using the Checkerboard DNA-DNA hybridization method, the microbial species adhered to toothbrush bristles after brushing and storage in different antimicrobial agents, for both closed and open containers.

STUDY I

IN VIVO EVALUATION OF THE EFFICACY OF ANTIMICROBIAL SOLUTIONS IN THE DISINFECTION OF DENTAL BRUSHES HELD IN A CLOSED CONTAINER

ABSTRACT: *In* this study, the effectiveness of different antimicrobial solutions in disinfecting toothbrushes was evaluated *in vivo.* The brushes were immersed in the tested solutions contained in closed plastic cases. Sixteen healthy, normotype volunteers (Process 2010.1.39.58.8) took part in a randomized, *crossover*, triple-blind, controlled clinical study in which three different solutions were used 1) Periogard® - 0.12% chlorhexidine gluconate; 2) Periobio® 0.12% chlorhexidine gluconate (test); 3) Cepacol® - Cetylpyridinium chloride 0.05% (test) and 4) sterilized tap water (positive control), one per week, were used to store the toothbrushes. The volunteers received a toothbrush and a standard dentifrice without any antimicrobial agent other than sodium fluoride. Each toothbrush was kept in a case with one of the solutions and evaluated for the presence or absence of microorganisms. After each stage, a seven-day *washout* period was observed and a new brush and solution were used. The samples were evaluated by microbial culture and DNA Checkerboard. The microbial culture tests showed bacterial contamination in the tap water, Periogard® and Cepacol® samples. Gram staining identified the following microorganisms: Gram-positive bacilli, Gram-negative bacilli, streptococci, molds and yeasts. Only one brush in the negative control group was contaminated with Gram-positive bacilli. It was concluded that the control group had a significantly higher total bacterial count than the test groups, with a higher prevalence of the species *P. micra*, *P. endodontalis*, *L. casei*, *P. putida*, *P. gingivalis*, *E. corrodens* and *E. faecalis* than the other solutions. The frequency of detection of contamination was the same for the two methods used and the antiseptics with the active ingredient chlorhexidine were more effective in decontaminating the brushes.

Keywords: Toothbrush; Bacterial contamination; Disinfection; Mouthwash; Closed cases.

PROPOSITION

The general objective of this clinical study was to evaluate the effectiveness of different antimicrobial solutions in disinfecting toothbrushes stored after use, immersed in a closed plastic case, compared to a control solution (sterilized tap water), using the Microbial Culture and DNA-Checkerboard methods.

MATERIAL AND METHODS

Selection of antimicrobial solutions

In this study, three antimicrobial solutions and a control solution were evaluated: 1. Periogard® (0.12% chlorhexidine gluconate); 2. Periobio® (0.12% chlorhexidine gluconate); Cepacol® (0.05% cetylpyridinium chloride) and sterilized tap water (positive control), Table 1.

Table 1. Rinses tested for disinfecting toothbrushes.

Code	Product	Manufacturer	Active ingredient
A	**Periogard®**	Colgate- Palmolive	Chlorhexidine gluconate 0.12%
B	**Periobio®**	Segmenta Farmacèutica Ltda.	Chlorhexidine gluconate 0.12% (test)
C	**Cepacol®**	Sanofi-Aventis Farmacèutica Ltda	Cetylpyridinium chloride 0.05% (test)
D	**Sterilized Tap Water**	LabDom/FORP*	Positive Control

*Molecular Dental Diagnosis Laboratory

Brush selection

Sixty-four (64) brushes of the same brand were used (Indicator® Interdental) purchased from the manufacturer Oral-B® , Size 35 soft, lote # 275042845, plus five brushes to check for contamination before first use (negative control), and a standardized toothpaste, as shown in Figure 1.

Picture. Oral-B® Indicator® Interdental toothbrush, (35 soft) and standard dentifrice.

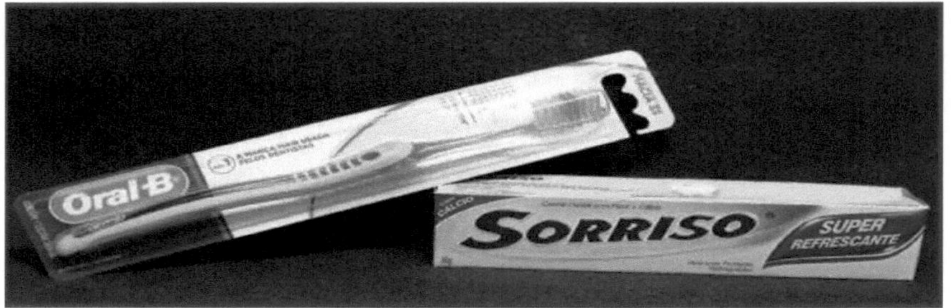

Selection of containers for the toothbrushes

Plastic containers with lids were used, purchased cheaply on the market and designated for food preservation purposes (approved for use in food preservation), as in Figure 2.

Figura 2. Plastic case for storing and disinfecting brushes.

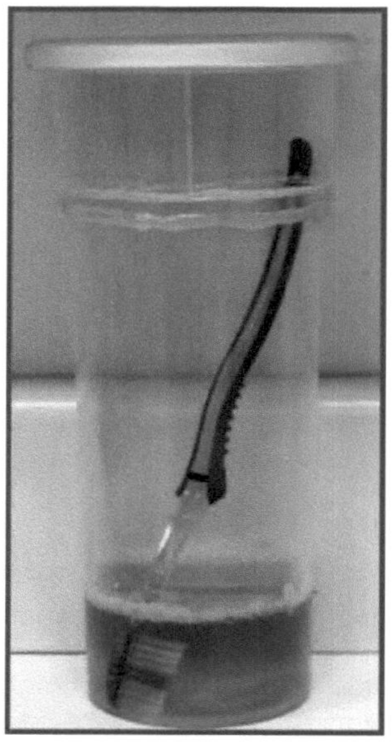

Patient selection

Sixteen patients (8 males and 8 females) in good health used all the solutions to be tested in a triple-blind (microbiologist, statistician and clinician), randomized controlled trial (RCT), designed as a *crossover*. The age range of the study subjects was between 18 and 30 years.

The participants met the following inclusion and exclusion criteria:

- Good general health;
- No signs of destructive periodontal disease;
- Minimum 24 teeth, six in each quadrant;
- Absence of antibiotic therapy (three months before the study);
- Non-smokers;
- No regular use of antiseptic mouthwashes;
- No use of corticoid therapy.

All the subjects received verbal and written instructions about the study in question and signed an informed consent form, approved by the Research Ethics Committee of FORP/USP (Process 2010.1.39.58.8). The individuals were divided into four groups, formed randomly by computer program (Excel spreadsheet, Windows Office 2003) with 4 members each. The groups used all types of solution, including the control, to preserve the toothbrushes in a closed case, in a *crossover* design.

Each research subject brushed their teeth three times a day (morning, after lunch and late afternoon) in the LabDom laboratory and was instructed to rinse their toothbrush with tap water after each use. The brushes were then stored individually in coded plastic cases (containers holding 200 mL of mouthwash or water) until their next use. Each stage lasted one week of storing the toothbrushes in daily use, and at the end of each clinical stage, a *washout* week was observed, a new toothbrush given to each participant and a new solution used by each participant to store the toothbrushes, until the cycle ended 7 weeks after the start of the clinical study. At the end of the clinical study, 4 brushes were used per subject, one for each disinfectant medium.

Sample preparation and microbiological processing.

All the microbiological steps were carried out in an aseptic environment, free from external contamination, in a laminar flow and with a Bunsen burner, in the facilities of the Molecular Dental Diagnostic Laboratory, following the protocol of Do Nascimento et al., 2011.

Evaluation of the negative control

Prior to the disinfection test, the negative control brushes were removed from their packaging to assess their possible contamination before use. The brushes were individually placed in test tubes with their heads immersed in 15 mL of peptone water culture medium (0.1% peptone, w/v). The tubes were incubated at 37°C for 14 days. At the end of the incubation period, aliquots of the culture medium were taken to confirm the presence of microorganisms using the microbial culture and DNA Checkerboad methods.

Brush disinfection test

After the brushing and storage period, the brushes were removed from the disinfection solutions and distilled water (control). A volume of 20 mL of each solution remaining in the storage jars was transferred to flasks containing 250 mL *of Letheen Broth* (Difco) and incubated at 37° C for up to 14 days. Microbial growth was observed by the presence of turbidity in the culture medium, and the day on which turbidity occurred was identified. If microorganisms grew and multiplied in the broth, aliquots of 500 µL were sown by serial dilution in Petri dishes to confirm contamination. The microorganisms contaminating the brushes were identified by microscopic morphology, using the Gram stain technique (Gram type, shape and grouping).

To assess contamination using the DNA Checkerboard hybridization method, 3 samples of 150 µL of each test solution were taken from each individual. The samples were neutralized with 150 µL of 0.5 M NaOH and stored at 4°C until processing.

RESULTS

The samples from the previous contamination test of the toothbrushes (negative control), as well as the samples of mouthwash and sterilized water used to store the toothbrushes during the experiment, were collected weekly and processed in the laboratory according to the protocols proposed in the Material and Methods section (Do Nascimento et al., 2011). Statistical analysis used the Kruskal-Wallis test for $p<0.05$ and Fisher's exact test.

Table 2 contains the results of the proportion of toothbrush contamination for each group studied, including the control (sterilized tap water), the bacterial counts and standard deviations (SD) of the 32 bacterial species collected from the containers containing the rinse solutions and tap water after 30 days of tooth brushing, obtained using the DNA-Checkerboard Technique.

Table 3 shows the number of samples detected or not as regards bacterial contamination, using the DNA-Checkerboard Hybridization or Bacterial Culture techniques. No significant differences were found by category using Fisher's Exact Test.

Figure 3 shows the average total bacterial count per group (x 10^5) and the standard error of the averages.

Table 2. Bacterial contamination of toothbrushes by group and standard deviation.

Species	H2O Proportion of contaminated samples	H2O Counting Bacterial (DP)	Periobio® Proportion of contaminated samples	Periobio® Counting Bacterial (DP)	Periogard® Proportion of contaminated samples	Periogard® Counting Bacterial (DP)	Cepacol Proportion of contaminated samples	Cepacol Counting Bacterial (DP)
S.mitis	0	0.00(0.00)	0	0.00(0.00)	0	0.00(0.00)	0	0.00(0.00)
S.gordonii	0	0.00(0.00)	0	0.00(0.00)	0	0.00(0.00)	0	0.00(0.00)
P.aeruginosa	0	0.00(0.00)	0	0.00(0.00)	0	0.00(0.00)	0	0.00(0.00)
N.mucosa	0	0.00(0.00)	0	0.00(0.00)	0	0.00(0.00)	0	0.00(0.00)
P.micra *	5/16	0.87(1.61)	0	0.00(0.00)	0	0.00(0.00)	0	0.00(0.00)
P.endodontalis **	6/16	0.48(0.72)	0	0.00(0.00)	0	0.00(0.00)	4/16	0.38(0.71)
L.casei **	7/16	0.67(1.00)	2/16	0.19(0.56)	3/16	0.26(0.58)	1/16	0.06(0.26)
Fperiodonticum	5/16	0.44(0.77)	2/16	0.09(0.27)	3/16	0.19(0.43)	1/16	0.05(0.22)
F.nucleatum	5/16	0.99(0.17)	1/16	0.04(0.18)	3/16	0.20(0.47)	0	0.00(0.00)
S.pasteuri	0	0.00(0.00)	0	0.00(0.00)	0	0.00(0.00)	0	0.00(0.00)
V.parvula	0	0.00(0.00)	1/16	0.02(0.10)	1/16	0.06(0.25)	1/16	0.05(0.21)
Tforsythia	3/16	0.12(0.28)	1/16	0.03(0.15)	0	0.00(0.00)	0	0.00(0.00)
T.denticola	0	0.00(0.00)	0	0.00(0.00)	0	0.00(0.00)	0	0.00(0.00)
S.moorei	1/16	0.03(0.13)	0	0.00(0.00)	0	0.00(0.00)	1/16	0.02(0.09)
S.parasanguinis	4/16	0.47(0.87)	1/16	0.05(0.23)	0	0.00(0.00)	4/16	0.16(0.33)
S.salivarius	4/16	0.60(0.11)	2/16	0.21(0.72)	1/16	0.06(0.26)	3/16	0.12(0.26)
S. sobrinus	3/16	0.06(0.15)	1/16	0.04(0.19)	0	0.00(0.00)	2/16	0.09(0.25)
S.sanguinis	1/16	0.01(0.07)	1/16	0.02(0.11)	0	0.00(0.00)	1/16	0.01(0.79)
S.oralis	3/16	0.29(0.78)	2/16	0.17(0.49)	0	0.00(0.00)	0	0.00(0.00)
S.mutans	1/16	0.0096 (0.03)	1/16	0.12(0.51)	0	0.00(0.00)	1/16	0.01(0.04)
S.constelatus	2/16	0.19(0.60)	0	0.00(0.00)	1/16	0.01(0.07)	2/16	0.18(0.58)
S.aureus	2/16	0.61(1.93)	0	0.00(0.00)	2/16	0.32(0.94)	0	0.00(0.00)
P.putida **	3/16	0.28(0.67)	0	0.00(0.00)	1/16	0.02(0.08)	0	0.00(0.00)
P.intermedia	1/16	0.02(0.10)	2/16	0.17(0.66)	2/16	0.13(0.44)	1/16	0.02(0.09)
Pmelaninogen	1/16	0.10(0.42)	2/16	0.09(0.27)	0	0.00(0.00)	1/16	0.03(0.15)
P.gingivalis **	5/16	1.11(1.82)	1/16	0.08(0.34)	1/16	0.02(0.09)	0	0.00(0.00)
E.corrodens **	4/16	0.55(1.02)	0	0.00(0.00)	0	0.00(0.00)	2/16	0.10(0.33)
Efaecalis **	5/16	0.46"(0.89)	1/16	0.03"(0.14)	0	0.00"(0.00)	1/16	0.02"(0.08)
C.gingivalis	1/16	0.03"(0.10)	1/16	0.07"(0.20)	0	0.00"(0.00)	1/16	0.01"(0.05)
B.fragillis	2/16	0.18"(0.50)	0	0.00"(0.00)	0	0.00"(0.00)	0	0.00"(0.00)
Aa a	3/16	0.33"(0.70)	0	0.00"(0.00)	0	0.00"(0.00)	0	0.00"(0.00)
Aa b	0	0.00"(0.00)	0	0.00"(0.00)	0	0.00"(0.00)	0	0.00"(0.00)

* Significant difference ($P < 0.01$; Friedman test)
** Significant difference ($P < 0.05$; Friedman test)

Table 3. Number of samples detected or not by the DNA-Checkerboard and Bacterial Culture Techniques.

	DNA Checkerboard				Culture				Total
	$H2O$	Periobio®	Periogard®	Cepacol®	$H2O$	Periobio®	Periogard®	Cepacol®	
Detection									
Yes	9	3	4	9	12	0	1	3	41
No	7	13	12	7	4	16	15	13	87
Total	16	16	16	16	16	16	16	16	128

No significant differences were found between the categories (Fisher's Exact Test).

Figura 3. Mean total bacterial count (x10[5] cells) and Standard Error of the mean in the 3 groups evaluated (*Difference detected by the Kruskal-Wallis test; $p<0.05$).

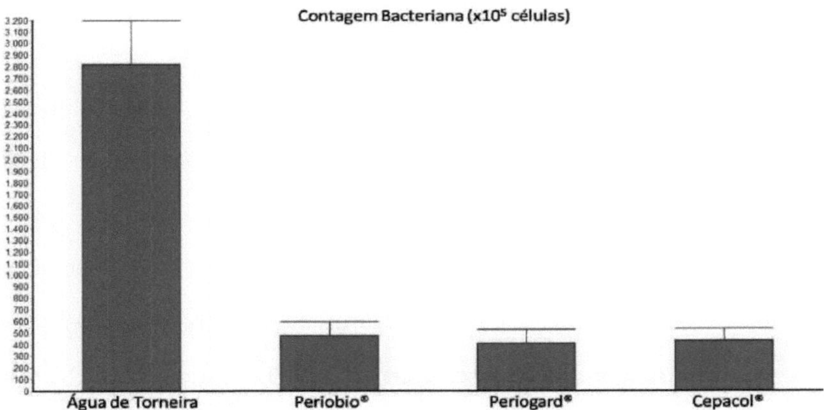

Statistical analysis.

The data obtained after the clinical stage were subjected to statistical analysis using parametric or non-parametric tests, depending on the distribution of the data.

DISCUSSION

Contemporary dentistry is increasingly taking a holistic approach to the primary and rehabilitative care of human beings. The "Theory of Focal Infection" has never been so current and with such repercussions in our daily lives, and at all levels of practice.

Many controversies accompany us in our daily clinical practice, where, for example, on the one hand we sterilize (sterilization, p.d. = destruction of all living forms) or at least disinfect (disinfection, p.d. = destruction of pathogens on inanimate surfaces) the entire arsenal to be used for a given dental treatment, seeking to maintain the aseptic chain by applying the BEDA system (barriers, sterilization, disinfection and antisepsis), doesn't it suggest a paradox that we use the toothbrush as the most commonly used instrument for sanitizing the soft and hard tissues of the mouth without taking any kind of precaution other than simply rinsing it after use?

The contamination of toothbrushes by microorganisms has been proven by several studies (Cobb, 1920; Dayoub et al., 1977; Svanberg, 1978; Marcano, 1981; Glass & Lare, 1986; Glass & Jensen, 1988; Müller et al., 1989; Malmberg et al., 1994; Carvajal et al., 1995; Borges et al, 1996; Verran & Leahy-Gilmartin, 1996; Hammond et al., 1997; Pinto et al., 1997; Taji & Rogers, 1998; Motzfeld et al., 1999; Long et al., 2000; Nelson Filho et al., 2000), and the presence of microorganisms has been observed not only in the oral cavity, but also in the environment in which they are stored. Thus, some way of eliminating these microorganisms would be desirable in order to avoid both re-infection of the patient and the occurrence of cross-contamination (Goh et al., 1985; Zarski & Leroy, 1999) through the "collective use" of the same toothbrush (Paschoal & Rotta, 1992; Bregagnolo et al., 1999; Grigoletto et al., 2000; Grigoletto et al., 2001).

Since simply rinsing the toothbrush, which is the generic method most commonly used by people, has proven to be ineffective (Glass & Lare, 1986; Kozai et al, 1989; Malmberg et al,

1994), various disinfection methods have been studied.

The solutions evaluated in this study were chosen to assess their ability to reduce microbial contamination on toothbrushes. A precaution taken to avoid subjectivism on the part of the laboratorian that could influence the results to be obtained was the numbering of the cases, so that there was no correspondence of numbers in the samples from the same individual. In this way, based on the result obtained in one week, the laboratory could not predict how many bacterial colonies would be found in the following weeks, since they didn't know which individual it came from.

CONCLUSIONS

Within the limitations of this study, it can be concluded that:

(1) When the bacterial count between the groups was carried out without distinguishing between the species evaluated, the control group (water) had a significantly higher count than the other groups (rinses);

(2) The species *P. micra*, *P. endodontalis*, *L. casei*, *P. putida*, *P. gingivalis*, *E. corrodens* and *E. faecalis* were found in higher counts in water compared to the other solutions;

(3) The frequency of contamination detection was the same for the two methods used;

(4) With regard to the negative contamination test, only one of the five brushes evaluated was contaminated by gram-positive bacilli;

(5) Antiseptics with the active ingredient chlorhexidine were more effective in decontaminating bacteria.

We would like to thank the **SÃO PAULO STATE RESEARCH FOUNDATION (FAPESP)** for the Scientific Initiation Scholarship awarded to **Maira Balero Sorgini**, a dentistry undergraduate student (process no. **2010/01292-7**).

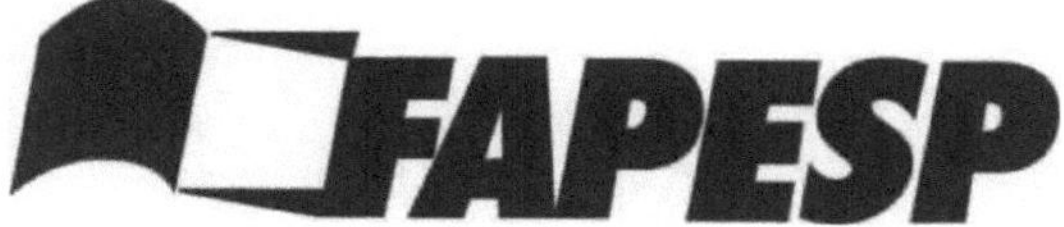

STUDY II

IN VIVO EVALUATION OF THE EFFECTIVENESS OF ANTIMICROBIAL SOLUTIONS IN DISINFECTING DENTAL BRUSHES HELD IN OPEN RECIPIENTS

ABSTRACT: The aim of this clinical investigation was to identify and quantify the microbial species adhered to the bristles of toothbrushes after supervised brushing and storage in different antimicrobial agents contained in open cases. Sixteen healthy participants were included in this study and randomized to four interventions in a crossover design: brushing and storage of toothbrushes in open cases containing: (I) Periogard® ; (II) Periobio® (chlorhexidine gluconate 0.12%); (III) Cepacol® (cetylpyridinium chloride 0.05%) and (IV) distilled water (positive control). Thirty-eight bacterial species, including putative pathogens and 5 *Candida spp.* were evaluated by the DNA hybridization technique DNA Checkerboard. Results: The results of the study showed a notable reduction in total microbial counts, including bacteria and *Candida spp.* on toothbrush bristles after storage in 0.05% cetylpyridinium chloride ($p < 0.0001$). Chlorhexidine gluconate at 0.12% showed no difference in total bacterial count when compared to distilled water ($p > 0.05$). Cetylpyridinium chloride solution also showed the lowest genome counts and frequency of detection for individual target species; distilled water showed the highest individual genome counts ($p < 0.05$). Potentially pathogenic species were recorded at moderate to high levels for chlorhexidine gluconate and distilled water. Conclusion: 0.05% cetylpyridinium chloride was the most effective storage solution in reducing total and individual microbial counts, including pathogenic species, when stored in open containers (cases).

Keywords: Toothbrush; Bacterial contamination; Disinfection; Mouthwash; Open cases.

PROPOSITION

Considering that microbial cell death can occur due to the absence of a significant amount of nutrients and/or microbial competition during the storage of toothbrushes, and that the products of cell lysis and degradation can interfere in the inflammatory process of oral tissues, we proposed in this randomized, controlled, cross-over study, controlled, cross-over study, a clinical evaluation with identification and quantification of microorganisms, using the Checkerboard DNA-DNA hybridization method, of the species adhered to toothbrush bristles after brushing and storage of toothbrushes in open containers (open cases) immersed in different antimicrobial agents. Thirty-eight bacterial species, including putative pathogens and 5 *Candida spp.* were investigated. Two hypotheses were tested: **antimicrobial solutions** (1) are capable of significantly reducing total microbial counts on bristles; (2) are effective in reducing pathogenic species.

MATERIAL AND METHODS

Selection of Antimicrobial Solutions

This study evaluated three mouthwashes commonly used as antimicrobial solutions for storing toothbrushes in open containers: chlorhexidine gluconate 0.12% (Periogard® ; Colgate-Palmolive Company, Sâo Paulo-SP, Brazil and Periobio® ; Segmenta Farmacêutica Ltda, Ribeirâo Preto-SP, Brazil); cetylpyridinium chloride 0.05% (Cepacol® - Sanofi-Aventis, Sâo Paulo-SP, Brazil). Sterile distilled water was used as a positive control for storing the toothbrushes, according to Table 1.

Table 1. Rinses tested for disinfecting toothbrushes.

Code	Product	Manufacturer	Active ingredient
A	**Periogard®**	Colgate- Palmolive	Chlorhexidine gluconate 0.12%
B	Periobio®	Segmenta Farmacèutica Ltda.	Chlorhexidine gluconate 0.12% (test)
C	**Cepacol®**	Sanofi-Aventis Farmacêutica Ltda	Cetylpyridinium chloride 0.05% (test)
D	**Sterilized Tap Water**	LabDom/FORP*	Positive Control

* Molecular Dental Diagnostic Laboratory

Brush and toothpaste selection

Sixty-four conventional toothbrushes (Oral-B Indicator® , Procter & Gamble Company, Sao Paulo-SP, Brazil) and a toothpaste containing sodium monofluorophosphate, 1500 ppm Flûor, calcium carbonate, sodium lauryl sulfate and sodium silicate (Kolynos do Brasil Ltda., Sao Bernardo do Campo, SP, Brazil) were used during brushing. All the toothbrush heads were similar in size, shape and number of regular bristles.

Selection of research subjects

Participants were selected from undergraduate students at the Ribeirao Preto School of Dentistry (University of Sao Paulo, Brazil). Sixteen healthy participants (8 men and 8 women; mean age (± SD) 20.33 ± 1.67 years) were recruited who had at least 28 teeth, no clinical signs of disease on the oral mucosa and healthy gums. Participants were not included if they were: pregnant or breastfeeding; had received periodontal treatment or antibiotics in the previous 3 months; smokers; had a systemic disease that could disturb the periodontium, or required pre-medication for dental treatment. In addition, an oral examination was carried out to ensure that all participants showed no signs or symptoms of pathological changes. The microbial cell count parameter was the primary variable for calculating the minimum sample size in this investigation, and this parameter was calculated using the PASS 2005 program (NCSS, Kaysville, USA). The reference standard deviations were taken from similar studies in the literature. The study was approved by the Research Ethics Committee of FORP/USP and all experiments were carried out with the written consent and acquiescence of each subject, in accordance with ethical principles (**CAAE 2010.1.1125.58.5**).

Experimental Design

All the participants enrolled in this research received oral hygiene instructions by means of an interactive presentation and an explanatory leaflet. They were instructed to brush their teeth 3 times a day (in the morning, in the middle of the day and in the late afternoon) for 7 days. They were advised to rinse their mouths with tap water after brushing. During the brushing period, the toothbrushes were stored individually in open containers containing 200 mL of one of the proposed solutions (**Periogard®**, **Periobio®**, **Cepacol®** or sterile distilled water). The containers were kept open throughout the experimental period. The participants received the following 4 interventions, according to a crossover design:

(I) Brushing and storing toothbrushes in **Periogard®**;

(II) Brushing and storing toothbrushes in Periobio®;

(III) Brushing and storing toothbrushes in Cepacol® e;

(IV) Brushing and storing toothbrushes in distilled water (positive control).

Each intervention was applied once and the results were evaluated after 7 days. The intervention sequence (I-II-II-IV) for each participant was obtained using computer-generated random numbers and hidden until the end of the data analysis. A 7-day *washout* period was followed between interventions. Hygiene instructions were applied again at the beginning of each intervention. All brushing and storage steps were carried out in the Molecular Dental Diagnosis Laboratory (LabDom) of the Department of Dental Materials and Prosthetics (Faculty of Dentistry of Ribeirâo Preto-USP, Brazil) under the supervision of an investigator. The study required a total of 7 weeks to complete the randomization and crossover project.

Microbiological sampling

Before tooth brushing, five toothbrushes were used as negative controls and evaluated to identify possible contamination of the bristles before contact with the oral cavity. All the toothbrush bristles from the negative controls and experimental interventions in each participant were removed from the head of the toothbrushes with a sterile scalpel blade and individually placed in microtubes containing 150 µL of TE solution (10 mM Tris-HCl, 1 mM EDTA, pH 8.0) followed by the addition of 150 µL of 0.5 M NaOH. The samples were stored at -20 °C until laboratory processing by Checkerboard DNA-DNA Hybridization. The total number of clinical samples after collection was 64 microtubes for experimental samples and 5 microtubes for the negative control.

Molecular Microbiological Evaluation

Microbial adherence on toothbrush bristles after brushing and storage in the proposed solutions was detected using the Checkerboard DNA-DNA hybridization molecular diagnostic method, according to Nascimento et al. (2010).

In this study, 38 bacterial species, including pathogenic and non-pathogenic microorganisms and 5 *Candida spp.* were selected for targeted detection during the investigation of microbial contamination of toothbrushes. Microbial species and their respective ATCC numbers are shown in Table 1.

Table 1 - Target species and ATCC reference number

Aggregatibacter actinomycetemcomitans serotype a	*29522*	*Pseudomonas putida*	12633
Aggregatibacter actinomycetemcomitans serotype b	29523	*Staphylococcus aureus*	25923
Bacteroides fragilis	25285	*Streptococcus constellatus*	27823
Capnocytophaga gingivalis	33624	*Streptococcus gordonii*	10558
Campylobacter rectus	33238	*Streptococcus mitis*	49456
Escherichia coli	10798	*Solobacterium moorei*	CCUG39336
Eikenella Corrodens	23834	*Streptococcus mutans*	25175
Enterococcus faecalis	51299	*Streptococcus oralis*	35037
Fusobacterium nucleatum	25586	*Streptococcus parasanguinis*	15911
Fusobacterium periodonticum	33693	*Staphylococcus pasteuri*	51129
Klebsiella pneumoniae	700721	*Streptococcus salivarius*	25975
Lactobacillus casei	393	*Streptococcus sanguinis*	10556
Mycoplasma salivarium	23064	*Streptococcus sobrinus*	27352
Neisseria mucosa	25996	*Tannerella forsythia*	43037
Pseudomonas aeruginosa	27853	*Treponema denticola*	35405
Peptostreptococcus anaerobius	49031	*Veillonella parvula*	10790
Porphyromonas endodontalis	35406		
Porphyromonas gingivalis	33277	*Candida albicans*	10231
Prevotella intermedia	25611	*Candida dubliniensis*	MYA 646
Prevotella melaninogenica	25845	*Candida glabrata*	90030
Parvimonas micra	33270	*Candida krusei*	6258
Prevotella nigrescens	33563	*Candida tropicalis*	750

Total genomic DNA probes from the 43 microbial species were directly labeled with the thermostable alkaline phosphatase enzyme using the AlkPhos Direct Marking and Detection System (GE Healthcare, UK). Briefly, 100 ng of denatured DNA was mixed with labeling buffer and alkaline phosphatase enzyme. Formaldehyde was then added to covalently cross-link the enzyme to the probe. The resulting alkaline phosphatase-labeled probes were adjusted to a final concentration of 1 ng/µL. Sensitivity and specificity tests were carried out for each labelled probe in order to optimize the amount of probe needed to detect 105 and 106 microbial cells of each species with the shortest possible history (SOKRANSKY et al., 2004).

For the microbiological evaluation of the clinical samples, microtubes containing bristles were boiled for 5 min to denature the DNA samples. The tubes were then immediately cooled on ice and the samples were mixed with 800 µL of 5 M ammonium acetate. The contents of each microtube were individually applied to a nylon membrane (Hybond N+, GE Healthcare Life Sciences do Brasil, Sâo Paulo-SP, Brazil) and cooked for 2 hours at 80 °C. As a standard reference, defined amounts of genomic DNA corresponding to 105 or 106 bacterial cells for each of the target species were also applied to the same set of membranes. The membranes were pre-hybridized at 60 °C for 2 hours in hybridization solution (0.5 M NaCl; 0.4% w/v blocking reagent).

After pre-hybridization, defined amounts of complete genomic probes labeled with the target species were applied individually to the samples concentrated on the membranes. The hybridization process was carried out overnight at 60 °C under gentle agitation. After washing, the hybridization signals were detected by chemiluminescence using CDP- Star (GE Healthcare) and the membranes were exposed to ECL Hyperfilm-MP (GE Healthcare).

Hyperfilm images were scanned and analyzed using TotalLab Quant software (TotalLab Ltd, Newcastle upon Tyne, UK).

DATA ANALYSIS

Total microbial counts and individuals (number of microbial cells adhered to the bristles) and prevalence (number of participants with positive detection for target species) were provided for all interventions tested. The number of microorganisms recovered from toothbrush bristles can be expressed in terms of counts by comparing the chemiluminescent intensity signals for samples and standard lines. To compare the microbial counts recovered from each intervention, the data were calculated under different experimental conditions. First, the microorganisms were analyzed individually and comparisons were made within a particular storage solution in order to differentiate the counts between the different target species; then, a specific target species was compared between different storage solutions. In a second analysis, the microorganisms were analyzed as a set of all 43 target species. Total microbial count data (including bacteria and *Candida spp.*), total bacterial count and total *Candida spp.* count were compared between the proposed interventions. Significant differences between the groups were calculated using Friedman's test followed by Dunn's post-test for multiple comparisons. The percentages of adherent microorganisms in the samples tested (prevalence) for each target species were also recorded. The two-way ANOVA test followed by the Bonferroni post-test was used to analyze the microbial detection frequencies for different storage solutions. Differences were considered significant when $p < 0.05$. GraphPad Prisma 5.0 statistical software (GraphPad Software Inc., La Jolla, CA, USA) was used for data analysis.

RESULTS

Individual Microbial Count

None of the samples used as a negative control showed positive signals for microbial detection. The prevalence and individual genome counts of the 43 target species found adhered to the bristles of the toothbrushes of the control (distilled water IV) and experimental (I, II and III) groups are presented as mean (x105 cells) and standard deviation (± SD). They are shown in Table 2.

Twenty-two out of 38 bacterial species and 3 out of 5 *Candida spp.*, including pathogenic and non-pathogenic species, showed significant differences in genomic counts between different storage solutions (Friedman's test followed by Dunn's post-test; $p < 0.05$). Overall, most of the target species were observed in reduced counts in group III and increased counts in the positive control (group IV).

Table 2 - Prevalence, microbial counts (x10[5] cells; ±SD) and respective p value for each target species after proposed interventions

Species	Cepacol			Periogard			Periobio			Distilled Water			
	Prevalence	Count	±SD	Prevalence	Count	±SD	Prevalence	Count	±SD	Prevalence	Count	±SD	p value
A. actinomycetencomitans	2/16	0.24	0.89	2/16	0.29	1.09	1/16	0.06	0.35	7/16	1.24	2.25	0.059
a	3/16	0.36	1.08	3/16	0.43	1.27	0/16	0	0	1/16	0.20	1.07	0.306
	7/16	0.87	1.55	3/16	0.57	1.42	1/16	0.06	0.36	5/16	0.73	1.62	0.198
	4/16	0.49	1.23	3/16	0.43	1.28	1/16	0.06	0.36	0/16	0	0	0.057
C.	0/16	0	0	4/16	0.59	1.48	1/16	0.07	0.40	0/16	0	0	0.0351
E. faecalis rectus	3/16	0.38	1.12	0/16	0	0	1/16	0.07	0.37	1/16	0.08	0.46	0.283
F. nucleatum E.	2/16	0.24	0.88	2/16	0.28	1.04	1/16	0.06	0.35	0/16	0	0	0.391
corrodens	4/16	0.51	1.27	4/16	0.71	1.56	0/16	0	0	0/16	0	0	0.0111
K. pneumoniae	2/16	0.24	0.91	3/16	0.42	1.25	1/16	0.06	0.36	0/16	0	0	0.0452
L. casei F.	4/16	0.61	1.54	3/16	0.56	1.42	1/16	0.06	0.36	0/16	0	0	0.129
M. salivarius periodonticum	2/16	0.31	1.15	5/16	0.85	1.66	1/16	0.06	0.36	0/16	0	0	0.0089
N. mucosa	4/16	0.56	1.40	5/16	0.85	1.67	0/16	0	0	2/16	0.21	0.80	0.083
	1/16	0.13	0.72	11/1	1.69	2.17	0/16	0	0	0/16	0	0	<0.0001
	5/16	0.70	1.58	9/16	1.67	2.36	0/16	0	0	0/16	0	0	*0.0002
P.	4/16	0.65	1.72	3/16	0.43	1.26	0/16	0	0	2/16	0.35	1.34	0.273
aeruginosa	3/16	0.44	1.30	14/1	2.23	2.31	1/16	0.05	0.34	0/16	0	0	<0.0001
anaerobios	2/16	0.29	1.10	13/1	2.16	2.43	1/16	0.07	0.40	3/16	0.55	1.67	*0.0001
endodontalis	4/16	0.66	1.67	9/16	1.48	2.03	1/16	0.07	0.38	0/16	0	0	*0.0004
gingivalis	2/16	0.26	0.95	8/16	1.30	1.92	2/16	0.15	0.58	2/16	0.24	0.92	0.0015
intermedia	5/16	0.82	1.66	1/16	0.14	0.76	2/16	0.15	0.57	3/16	0.53	1.64	0.171
melaninogenica	5/16	0.57	1.46	4/16	0.56	1.41	2/16	0.18	0.69	5/16	0.84	1.92	0.373
micra	6/16	0.85	1.70	2/16	0.28	1.04	2/16	0.15	0.57	2/16	0.33	1.23	0.208
nigrescens	4/16	0.57	1.44	12/1	1.86	2.21	3/16	0.30	0.92	0/16	0	0	0.0002
putida	7/16	0.98	1.75	2/16	0.24	1.04	0/16	0	0	2/16	0.41	1.51	0.0257
aureus	2/16	0.43	1.28	1/16	0.14	0.75	0/16	0	0	0/16	0	0	0.111
constelatus	1/16	0.14	0.76	9/16	1.31	1.95	1/16	0.07	0.38	0/16	0	0	<0.0001
gordonii	5/16	0.68	1.50	8/16	1.31	1.93	2/16	0.15	0.57	4/16	0.74	1.97	*0.0149
mitis	5/16	0.63	1.39	7/16	1.15	1.86	1/16	0.07	0.37	9/16	1.18	1.82	0.0186
moreei	5/16	0.63	1.39	6/16	0.86	1.69	2/16	0.15	0.57	10/1	1.43	2.11	0.0009
mutans	5/16	0.66	1.45	10/1	1.46	2.00	3/16	0.27	0.83	12/1	1.83	2.38	0.0009
oralis	5/16	0.64	1.41	10/1	1.46	2.00	1/16	0.08	0.42	4/16	0.67	1.70	0.0018
parasanguinis	3/16	0.38	1.13	5/16	0.71	1.55	1/16	0.08	0.42	6/16	0.86	1.78	0.107
pasteuri	4/16	0.51	1.27	2/16	0.42	1.26	1/16	0.07	0.40	8/16	1.06	1.77	0.050
salivarius	2/16	0.26	0.97	9/16	1.39	2.07	2/16	0.16	0.59	1/16	0.09	0.50	0.0019
S. sobrinus saguinis	1/16	0.13	0.69	5/16	0.78	1.71	2/16	0.16	0.59	15/1	2.82	2.89	<0.0001
T. forshytia	5/16	0.63	1.38	0/16	0	0	3/16	0.24	0.71	2/16	0.27	1.00	*0.157
T.	8/16	1.29	2.24	0/16	0	0	1/16	0.09	0.51	16/1	3.31	3.03	<0.0001
denticola	6/16	0.78	1.55	1/16	0.14	0.75	2/16	0.07	0.37	16/1	2.90	2.97	*0.0001
parvula	6/16	0.78	1.53	5/16	0.87	1.69	0/16	0	0	13/1	1.88	2.16	*0.0040
albicans	3/16	0.39	1.17	3/16	0.28	1.04	1/16	0.07	0.39	9/16	0.68	1.29	0.063
dubliniensis	4/16	0.49	1.23	4/16	0.57	1.43	3/16	0.25	0.75	8/16	0.98	1.61	0.161
glabrata	8/16	1.12	1.88	10/1	1.65	2.10	0/16	0	0	16/1	3.05	2.73	<0.0001
krusei tropicalis 16/16	13/15	1.99	2.38	6 11/15	1.69	2.15	1/16	0.06	0.36	6	3.32	3.53	*0.0001

*Differences in a particular species bewteen different solutions detected by Friedman test followed by Dunn's multiple comparisons post-tests ($p<0.05$)

When a given species was compared within the same storage solution, *Candida tropicalis* was the only species that showed significant differences in group I, with the highest genome count (1.99 ± 2.38; p = 0.0084). In group II, 6 species showed significant differences (p <0.0001). *Escherichia coli, Tanerella forsythia and Treponema denticola* were not detected in any of the participants; and *Peptostreptococcus anaerobius* (2.23 ± 2.31), *Porphyromonas endodontalis* (2.16 ± 2.43) and *Pseudomonas putida* (1.86 ± 2.21) had the highest genome counts. No significant differences were observed in the genome counts of the target species when the brushes were stored in solution III (p = 0.8961), which had the lowest individual genome counts. In group IV (distilled water), *Streptococcus sobrinus* (2.82 ± 2.89), *T. denticola* (3.31 ± 3.03), *Veillonella parvula* (2.90 ± 2.97), *Candida krusei* (3.05 ± 2.73) and *C. tropicalis* (3.32 ± 3.53) had the highest genome counts (p <0.0001).

Microbial prevalence

When the target species were evaluated as a set of microorganisms, all the storage solutions tested showed significant differences detected by the Friedman test, followed by Dunn's multiple comparisons after the tests (p <0.0001). Group III had the lowest average percentage (%, ± SD) of microorganisms adhered to the bristles (0.07 ± 0.05) when compared to groups I (0.25 ± 0.14); II (0.33 ± 0.24) and IV (0.28 ± 0.33), which showed no significant differences between them (p> 0.05). The prevalence of each target species in the proposed interventions is summarized in Table 2. All the storage solutions showed significant differences according to the Two-way ANOVA test and Bonferroni post-test (p<0.0001). Overall, Cepacol® showed the lowest percentages of pathogenic species related to periodontal diseases (*P. gingivalis, T. forsythia, T. denticola* and *Aggregatibacter actinomycetencomitans* - serotypes a and b), caries (*Streptococcus spp.) and* stomatitis (*Candida spp.*).

DISCUSSION

In this study, we used the Checkerboard DNA-DNA hybridization method to identify and quantify the microbial species adhered to the bristles of toothbrushes after controlled brushing and storage in different antimicrobial agents. In addition, we evaluated the effectiveness of the storage solutions in reducing pathogenic species. Thirty-eight bacterial species, including putative pathogens and 5 *Candida spp.* were investigated. The results of the study showed a notable reduction in total microbial counts, including bacteria and *Candida spp.* on toothbrush bristles after storage in 0.05% cetylpyridinium chloride. Chlorhexidine gluconate 0.12% showed no difference in the total bacterial count when compared to distilled water (positive control). However, chlorhexidine gluconate was effective in reducing the total *Candida spp.* With regard to the evaluation of individual microbial counts, toothbrushes stored in cetylpyridinium chloride solution also showed the lowest genome counts and frequency of detection for individual target species. Samples recovered from distilled water had the highest individual genome counts. Potentially pathogenic species were recorded at moderate to high levels for chlorhexidine gluconate and distilled water.

There are several studies in which the effectiveness of toothbrush disinfection on microbial colonization of the bristles is reported (KOMIYAMA et al., 2010; NELSON-FILHO et al., 2011; CHAMELE et al., 2012; PEKER et al., 2014), most of which were carried out by in vitro analyses. There are more published studies on the disinfection of toothbrushes using in vivo analyses, in which microbial colonization is measured. However, most of these studies were carried out using culture-based methods and only a few species of microorganisms were evaluated, most often those related to non-demanding species (SATO et al., 2005; NELSON-FILHO 2006 and 2013).

Overall, the mean microbial count values were higher in our study when compared to the literature. Culture-independent methods, such as the Checkerboard DNA-DNA hybridization method used in this study, can detect viable and non-viable microorganisms and can provide substantial information about the presence of non-culturable and/or fastidious species adhered to toothbrush bristles. In addition, these methods are faster and more suitable than traditional culture methods (SOCRANSKY et al., 2004).

According to the results of our study, high levels of non-pathogenic and pathogenic microorganisms were found adhering to the bristles after brushing and storing the toothbrushes in distilled water. These findings were expected and are in line with those reported by Sato et al. (2005) and Nelson-Filho et al. (2013) who observed, using culture methods, high levels of *Sreptococcus mutans* contamination on toothbrushes used by children and adults, which corroborates those reported by do Nascimento et al, (2014) using DNA hybridization analysis, in which several species of microorganisms were detected colonizing adult toothbrushes.

Similar to the findings reported in the literature, the storage of toothbrushes in antimicrobial agents in the present study significantly reduced the total microbial count and the individual genome count for most of the target species (KOMIYAMA et al., 2010; PEKER et al., 2014 and NELSON-FILHO et al. (2006). However, unlike most of these studies, cetylpyridinium chloride was the most effective antiseptic for individual and total microbial counts, including periodontopathogenic species, and not chlorhexidine gluconate. These data are not surprising, as cetylpyridinium chloride has been extensively reported as an effective antimicrobial agent, reducing biofilm formation, biofilm microbial colonization and gingival inflammation parameters (do NASCIMENTO et al, 2014; NELSON-FILHO et al., 2013; HAPS et al., 2008; HERRERA et al., 2009; VAN LEEUWEN et al., 2015). This agent is a quaternary ammonium whose antibacterial activity is the result of inactivation of energy-producing enzymes, denaturation of essential proteins and rupture of the cell membrane.

Cetylpyridinium chloride has been reported to be effective on Gram-positive and Gram-negative microorganisms, as well as fungi (GIULIANA et al., 1997).

A novelty of this research in relation to studies evaluating toothbrush contamination was the use of DNA-DNA Checkerboard hybridization for microbial detection and identification. This method allows the rapid and simultaneous identification of several microbial species (up to 45) in a large number (up to 28) of oral samples. In addition, the possibility of including difficult-to-cultivate, uncultivated or uncharacterized species in the set of target species can lead to a more comprehensive investigation of microorganism communities in oral infections (SOCRANSKY et al., 2004).

A possible explanation for the differences between the microbial counts in our study when compared to other similar investigations in the literature may be related to the sensitivity of the method used, which allows the detection of non-viable microorganisms in addition to viable ones. In our study, we were able to detect and identify viable and non-viable cells. This could explain the higher levels of contamination in our data when compared to culture-based studies (SATO et al., 2005; NELSON-FILHO et al., 2014). This could also be a reason for the higher count of microorganisms in the chlorhexidine gluconate groups when compared to cetylpyridinium chloride. Perhaps, most of the species detected in the chlorhexidine group may have died as a result of the antimicrobial agent, but their genetic material may be preserved, reflecting the positive detection.

These results may suggest that cetylpyridinium chloride can cause cell death and degradation of genetic material. However, further studies are needed to investigate these findings and the potential impact of dead microorganisms and/or their cell lysis products on clinical outcomes. Cell death with consequent DNA degradation by the proteolytic enzymes bactericin and endonucleases was demonstrated by Cascales et al., 2007.

An additional longitudinal study, using the same experimental protocol and evaluating clinical parameters, could provide more evidence on this issue. Conventional culture methods can also be applied in conjunction with molecular methods to assess the viability of target species.

CONCLUSIONS

Within the limitations of this research, the results of the study confirmed the hypotheses tested:

(1) cetylpyridinium chloride 0.05% was effective in reducing total microbial counts (including bacteria and *Candida spp.*) on toothbrush bristles; chlorhexidine gluconate 0.12% was effective in reducing total *Candida spp.* counts, but showed no difference in total bacterial counts when compared to distilled water;

(2) toothbrush bristles stored in cetylpyridinium chloride also showed the lowest microbial counts and frequency of detection for the individual target species, including pathogens.

Pathogenic species were recorded at moderate to high levels for chlorhexidine gluconate and distilled water.

REFERENCES*[1]

AAS JA, PASTER BJ, STOKES LN, OLSEN I, DEWHIRST FE. Defining the Normal Bacterial Flora of the Oral Cavity. **J Clin Microbiol** 2005; 43(11)5721-5732.

BOGOPOLSKY S. **La brosse à dents** (L'histoire de la "mal aimée"). Paris: Éditions CdP, 1995. 101p.

BONESVOLL, P.; GJERMO, P. A comparison between chlorhexidine and some quaternary ammonium compounds with regard to retention, salivary concentration and plaque-inhibiting effect in the human mouth after mouth rinses. **Arch. Oral Biol**. 1978;23(4):289-94.

CASCALES E, BUCHANAN SK, DUCHÉ D, KLEANTHOUS C, LLOUBÈS R, POSTLE K, et al. Colicin biology. **Microbiol Mol Biol** Rev 2007;71:158-229.

CAUDRY SD, KLITORINOS A, CHAN EC. Contaminated toothbrushes and their disinfection. **J Can Dent Assoc**. 1995;61(6):511-6.

CHAMELE J, BHAT C, SARAF T, JADHAV A, BEG A, JAGTAP C, et al. Efficacy of microwaves and chlorhexidine for disinfection of pacifiers and toothbrushes: an in vitro study. **J Contemp Dent Pract** 2012;13(5):690-694.

COBB CM. Toothbrushes as a cause of repeated infections of the mouth. **Boston Med. Surg. J.** 1920;183:263-264.

CROCOMBE LA, BRENNAN DS, SLADE GD, LOC DO. Is self interdental cleaning associated with dental plaque levels, dental calculus, gingivitis and periodontal disease? **J Periodontal Res** 2012;47(2):188-197.

DAJANI AS et al. Prevention of bacterial endocarditis. Recommendations by the American Heart Association. **JAMA**, 1990;264:2919-2922.

Do NASCIMENTO C et al. The use of fluorescein for labeling genomic probes in the checkerboard

*[1]According to: International Committee of Medial Joumal Editors - ANSI standard, adapted by the U.S. National Library of Medicine (VANCOUVER style). Available at: http://www.ncbi.nlm.nih.gov/bookshelf/br.fcgi?book=citmed (accessed October 15, 2017).

DNA-DNA hybridization method. **Microbiol Res**. 2008;163(4):403-7.

do NASCIMENTO C, de ALBUQUERQUE RF Jr, MONESI N, CANDIDO-SILVA JA. Alternative method for direct DNA probe labeling and detection using the checkerboard hybridization format. **J Clin Microbiol** 2010;48(8):3039-3040.

do NASCIMENTO C, SCARABEL TT, MIANI PK, WATANABE E, PEDRAZZI V. *In vitro* evaluation of the microbial contamination on new toothbrushes: A preliminary study. **Microscopy Research and Technique (Print)**, -epub *ahead of print*, 2011.

FRAZELLE MR, MUNRO CL. Toothbrush contamination: a review of the literature. **Nurs Res Pract** 2012;2012:420630.

GLASS RT, LARE MM. Toothbrush contamination: a potential health risk? **Quintessence Int.** 1986;17(1):39-42.

GENDREAU L, LOEWY ZG. Epidemiology and etiology of denture stomatitis. **J Prosthodont** 2011;20(4):251-260.

GIULIANA G, PIZZO G, MILICI ME, MUSOTTO GC, GIANGRECO R. In vitro antifungal properties of mouthrinses containing antimicrobial agents. **J Periodontol** 1997;68(8):729-733.

GOHLER A, HETZER A, HOLTFRETER B, GEISEL MH, SCHMIDT CO, STEINMETZ I, et al. Quantitative molecular detection of putative periodontal pathogens in clinically healthy and periodontally diseased subjects. **PLoS One** 2014;9(7):e99244.

GOLDING, P. S. The development of the toothbrush: A short story of tooth cleansing. Part 1: **Dent. Health.** 1982;21(4):25-7.

GUPTA G, MITRA D, ASHOK KP, GUPTA A, SONI S, AHMED S, et al. Efficacy of preprocedural mouth rinsing in reducing aerosol contamination produced by ultrasonic scaler: a pilot study. **J Periodontol** 2014;85(4):562-568.

HAPS S, SLOT DE, BERCHIER CE, VAN DER WEIJDEN GA. The effect of cetylpyridinium chloride-containing mouth rinses as adjuncts to toothbrushing on plaque and parameters of gingival inflammation: a systematic review. **Int J Dent Hyg** 2008;6(4):290-303.

HERRERA D. Cetylpyridinium chloride-containing mouth rinses and plaque control. **Evid Based Dent** 2009;10(2):44.

IȘERI U, ULUDAMAR A, OZKAN YK. Effectiveness of different cleaning agents on the adherence of Candida albicans to acrylic denturebase resin. **Gerodontology** 2011;28(4):271-276.

KANNER L. Folklore of the teeth. VII. The folklore and cultural history of the toothpick and toothbrush. **Dental Cosmos**. 1926;68(7):691-701.

KAUFFMAN JH. A study of the toothbrush. **Dental Cosmos**, Philadelphia, v.66, n.3, p.300-13, 1924.

MARCANO C. The toothbrush in the ecology of *Candida albicans*. **Mycopathologia**, 1981;74(3):135-41.

KETTERING JD. An *in vitro* investigation of the efficacy of CPC for use in toothbrush decontamination. **J Dent Hyg**. 1996;70(4):161-5.

KOLENBRANDER PE, LONDON J. Adhere today, here tomorrow: oral bacterial adherence. **J Bacteriol** 1993;175(11):3247-3252.

KOLENBRANDER PE. Oral microbial communities: biofilms, interactions, and genetic systems. **Annu Rev Microbiol** 2000;54:413-437.

KOLENBRANDER PE, PALMER JR RJ, PERIASAMY S, JAKUBOVICS NS. Oral multispecies biofilm development and the key role of cell-cell distance. **Nat Rev Microbiol** 2010; 8(7):471-80.

KOMIYAMA EY, Back-Brito GN, Balducci I and Koga-Ito CY. Evaluation of alternative methods for the disinfection of toothbrushes. Braz Oral Res 2010;24(1):28-33.

KOWALSKI J, GÓRSKA R. Clinical and microbiological evaluation of biofilm-gingival interface classification in patients with generalized forms of periodontitis. **Pol J Microbiol** 2014;63(2):175-81.

LEONHARDT A, BERGSTROM C, LEKHOLM U. Microbiologic diagnostics at titanium implants. **Clin Implant Dent Relat Res** 2003;5(4):226-232.

MARCANO C. El cepillo de dientes en la ecologia *de Candida albicans*. **Mycopathologia**. 1981;74(3):135-41.

MARSH PD. Plaque as a biofilm: pharmacological principles of drug delivery and action in the sub-

and supragingival environment. **Oral Diseases**, 2003; 9(Suppl 1): 16-22.

MAYANAGI G, SATO T, SHIMAUCHI H, TAKAHASHI N. Detection frequency of periodontitis-associated bacteria by polymerase chain reaction in subgingival and supragingival plaque of subjects with periodontitis and healthy subjects. **Oral Microbiol Immunol** 2004;19(6):379-385.

MEIER S, COLLIER C, SCALETTA MG, STEPHENS J, KIMBROUGH R,

McCAULEY, HB. Toothbrushes, toothbrush materials and design. **J. Am. Dent. Assoc.** 1946;33(5):283-93.

MELVILLE TH. Bacteria on the toothbrush. **Br. Dent. J.** 1961;111(3):90-2.

MEHTA A, SEQUEIRA PS, BHAT G. Bacterial contamination and decontamination of toothbrushes after use. **N Y State Dent J**. 2007;73(5):12-3.

NELSON FILHO P, MACARI S, FARIA G, ASSED S, ITO IY. Microbial contamination of toothbrushes and their decontamination. **Pediatr. Dent.** 2000;22(5):381-4.

NELSON-FILHO P, FARIA G, DA SILVA RA, ROSSI MA, ITO IY. Evaluation of the contamination and disinfection methods of toothbrushes used by 24- to 48-month-old children. **J Dent Child** 2006;73(3):152-158.

NELSON-FILHO P, DA SILVA LA, DA SILVA RA, ITO IY et al. Efficacy of microwaves and chlorhexidine on the disinfection of pacifiers and toothbrushes: an in vitro study. **Pediatr Dent** 2011;33(1):10-13.

NELSON-FILHO P, PEREIRA MS, DE ROSSI A et al. Children's toothbrush contamination in day-care centers: how to solve this problem? **Clin Oral Investig** 2014 Nov;18(8):1969-74.

NIKITKOVA AE, HAASE EM, SCANNAPIECO FA. Taking the Starch out of Oral Biofilm Formation: Molecular Basis and Functional Significance of Salivary α-Amylase Binding to Oral Streptococci. **Appl Environ Microbiol** 2013;79(2): 416-423.

OVERMAN PR. Biofilm: A New View of Plaque. **The Journal of Contemporary Dental Practice**. 2000; 1:1-8.

PADER M. **Oral hygiene products and practice**. New York: Marcel Dekker, 1988. 543p.

PEKER I, AKCA G, SARIKIR C, ALKURT MT, CELIK I. Effectiveness of alternative methods for toothbrush disinfection: an in vitro study. **Scientific World Journal** 2014;2014:726190.

PINTO EDR, PAIVA EMM, PIMENTA FC. Viability of anaerobic microorganisms from the oral cavity on toothbrushes. **Periodontia**, 1997;6(1):8-12.

RAMAGE G, CULSHAW S, JONES B, WILLIAMS C. Are we any closer to beating the biofilm: novel methods of biofilm control. **Curr Opin Infect Dis** 2010;23(6):560-6.

RING, M. E. **Dentistry**: an illustrated history. New York: Harry N. Abrams, 1985. 320p.

SAMSON E. The problem of the toothbrush. **Community Health**, 1972;3(5):226-30.

SCONYERS JR, CRAWFORD JJ, MORIARTY JD. Relationship of bacteremia to toothbrushing in patients with periodontitis. **J. Am. Dent. Assoc.** 1973;87(3):616-22.

SATO S, ITO IY, LARA EHG, PANZERI H, ALBUQUERQUE JÛNIOR RF, PEDRAZZI V. Bacterial survival rate on toothbrushes and their decontamination with antimicrobial solutions. **Journal of Applied Oral Science**, 2004;12(2):99-103.

SATO S, PEDRAZZI V, PANZERI H, LARA EHG, ITO IY. Antimicrobial spray for toothbrush disinfection: an in vivo evaluation. **Quintessence International**, 2005;36(10):812-6.

SOCRANSKY SS, HAFFAJEE AD, SMITH C, MARTIN L, HAFFAJEE JA, UZEL NG, et al. Use of checkerboard DNA-DNA hybridization to study complex microbial ecosystems. **Oral Microbiol Immunol** 2004;19(6):352-362.

SPOLIDORIO DMP, GOTO E, NEGRINI TDC, SPOLIDORIO LC. Viability of Streptococcus mutans on transparent and opaque toothbrushes. **J Dent Hyg** 2003;77(2):114-117.

SVANBERG M. Contamination of toothpaste and toothbrush by *Streptococcus mutans*. **Scand. J. Dent. Res.** 1978;86(5):412-4.

TEN CATE JM, MARSH PD. Procedures for establishing efficacy of antimicrobial agents for chemotherapeutic caries prevention. **J Dent Res** 1994;73(3):695-703.

TEN CATE, JACOB M. Biofilms, a new approach to the microbiology of dental plaque. **Odontology** 2006;94:1-9.

TAKAHASHI N. Microbial ecosystem in the oral cavity: Metabolic diversity in an ecological niche and its relationship with oral diseases. International Congress Series 2005;1284:103-112.

TAWAKOLI PN, AL-AHMAD A, HOTH-HANNIG W, HANNIG M, HANNIG C. Comparison of different live/dead stainings for detection and quantification of adherentmicroorganisms in the initial oral biofilm. **Clin Oral Investig**. 2013 Apr;17(3):841-50.

VAN LEEUWEN M, ROSEMA N, VERSTEEG P, SLOT D, VAN WINKELHOFF A, VAN DER WEIJDEN G. Long-term efficacy of a 0.07% cetylpyridinium chloride mouth rinse in relation to plaque and gingivitis: a 6-month randomized, vehicle-controlled clinical trial. **Int J Dent Hyg** 2015 May;13(2):93-103.

XU X, HE J, XUE J, WANG Y, LI K, ZHANG K, et al. Oral cavity contains distinct niches with dynamic microbial communities. **Environ Microbiol**. 2015 Mar;17(3):699- 710.

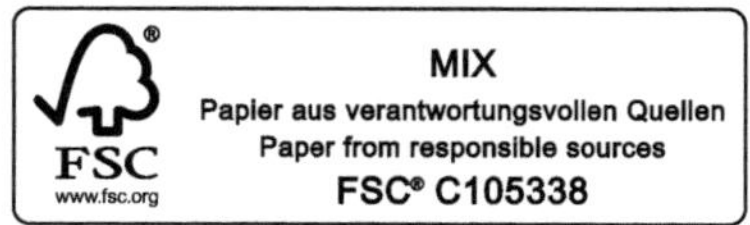

Printed by Books on Demand GmbH, Norderstedt / Germany